I0407808

Intermittent Fasting

The complete guide to permanent fat loss, lean muscle and healthy living

Daniel Jonas

Respective authors own all copyrights not held by the publisher.

The information herein is offered for informational purposes solely, and is universal as so. The presentation of the information is without contract or any type of guarantee assurance.

The trademarks that are used are without any consent, and the publication of the trademark is without permission or backing by the trademark owner. All trademarks and brands within this book are for clarifying purposes only and are the owned by the owners themselves, not affiliated with this document.

Table of Contents

Introduction

Thank you and congratulations for downloading *Intermittent Fasting: The complete guide to permanent fat loss, lean muscle and healthy living.*

Here is a shocking fact: According to World Health Organization, there are around a total of one billion adults who are overweight in the world today, and of those one billion adults, at least 300 million are said to be clinically obese. That's how alarming the rate of obesity has got, which is heartbreaking considering the numerous chronic conditions that come with it.

If you are overweight or you feel like you're heading there, then this book is for you. This book is going to teach you about intermittent fasting, which is one of the best methods that you can use to lose weight. The good thing about intermittent fasting is that it not only helps you lose weight but also helps you boost your metabolism as well as build lean muscles.

In this book, you will learn how intermittent fasting works, why it's the best option for weight loss, and the types of intermittent fasting that you can use to manage your cravings and lose weight.

Thank you once again for having a personal copy of this book. Enjoy!

Intermittent Fasting: What It Is and How It Works

Intermittent fasting is an eating pattern that involves cycling between periods of fasting and eating. With intermittent fasting, you make a conscious decision of skipping certain meals during the day. By doing so, you end up restricting your calorie intake, which leads to increased weight loss and lean body.

How Intermittent Fasting Works

In order to understand how intermittent fasting works, you need to know what happens when you eat normally. Most of us take at least three meals a day: breakfast, lunch, and dinner. It is what we were taught, and it was how we were raised.

After every single meal that you take, your body normally breaks down the food into glucose, which is its main source of energy. The presence of glucose in your bloodstream automatically triggers the production of insulin, which transports it to tissues and cells for energy provision.

During that process, two interesting things happen to your body. First, since insulin only concentrates on helping your body use glucose for energy, your body does not break down any stored fat for energy as long as there is glucose.

Secondly, insulin automatically stores any excess glucose after transportation as fat. Insulin basically encourages fat storage for the purpose of it being used later when your body is low on energy. The problem with this concept is that with three meals per day, your body hardly experiences the low energy levels that are usually supposed to force it into burning the fat store for energy. So, what happens is that your body constantly stores fat, which automatically leads to weight gain.

So, what happens with intermittent fasting that helps you lose weight?

Throughout history, human beings have been practicing fasting. Our ancestors were fasting experts who used to feast in times of plenty and fast in times of scarcity. Throughout their lives, they never experienced problems like obesity and chronic diseases. What intermittent fasting does to you is that it helps you change your eating lifestyle to that of your ancestors, which made them lean and healthy.

To understand how intermittent fasting works, you must first know the difference between the fed state, the post-absorptive state, and the fasted state. When you eat your meal, your body automatically gets into a fed state (a state where you are digesting and absorbing your food). This state normally starts from the minute you start eating and lasts for 3–5 hours. In the fed state, your body is normally high on insulin, which means it only burns glucose for energy.

After 5 hours, your body enters into the post-absorptive state where it doesn't process any meal. This state normally lasts for 8–12 hours after your last meal.

After 12 hours, your body now enters into a fasted state, which is where the magic happens. In the fasted state, your body reaches a point where it needs energy but there is no glucose for it to absorb as energy. This forces the body to start burning stored fats for energy, which automatically leads to weight loss.

Basically, what intermittent fasting does is that it sets aside some time for you to eat whatever you want and then alternate that with some fasting times that force your body to burn fat for energy. In short, intermittent fasting is a fat-burning machine that makes sure you are constantly burning the stored fat that causes weight gain.

However, why choose intermittent fasting?

Why Intermittent Fasting?

In the world today, there are numerous of ways that you can use to lose weight. But, why should you choose intermittent fasting over all those others?

This chapter is going to show you why intermittent fasting stands out among other weight loss methods by highlighting the various benefits that come with it as it is more than just a weight loss program. Some benefits you stand to gain by practicing intermittent fasting are as follows.

Better Detoxification

This may come to you as a surprise, but your body cleanses and detoxifies itself on a daily basis. Millions of cellular processes go on in your body, and it is usually your body's duty to identify the worn-out cells and replace them. This process is commonly known as autophagy, and it is a normal process that happens constantly.

The ongoing process of autophagy is usually affected by two things. The first one is a bad diet, and the second one is frequent eating. Usually, when you eat, the process of autophagy is slowed down because your body changes its focus from cleansing and detoxifying to digestion and absorption.

If you take meals only a few hours (5–6 hours) apart from each other, your cleansing process normally slows down making you feel tired as the lack of repair will be taking a toll on your cells.

One of the advantages of intermittent fasting is that it gives your body time to focus on the process of cellular repair because it discourages constant eating and encourages long hours of fasting. Therefore, with intermittent fasting, you stand a chance of boosting your body's detoxification process.

Less Hunger

Intermittent fasting is considered one of the best ways to lose weight because it deals with the one thing that makes it difficult for people to follow a diet, hunger.

Intermittent fasting is known for managing hunger and appetite, which makes the process of losing weight easier and fun. But how does it do this? Intense hunger is usually caused by blood sugar fluctuations, especially when your diet is high in carbohydrates.

When you eat a high-carb meal, your body produces high levels of insulin to manage the sugar levels. Insulin encourages your body cells to use the energy, and the rest is stored as fat, and this leads to a sudden drop in blood sugar levels. This sends a message to your brain that you need to eat to maintain your blood sugar level and the cycle continues.

Intermitted fasting manages your appetite by controlling your hunger hormones. When you practice intermittent fasting, your body normally relies on stored fat for energy. When that happens, the fat cell produces a hormone called Leptin, which regulates the hunger hormone ghrelin. It does this by telling your brain to turn off the hunger signals from ghrelin, which makes you rarely feel hungry when you are fasting.

Lowered Risk of Type-2 Diabetes

One of the advantages of intermittent fasting is that it uses up all of the glucose in your body and starts using fat for energy. That process usually lowers your body's blood sugar levels, which in turn reduces your risk of getting type-2 diabetes.

According to a study that was done on intermittent fasting, it was found out that the blood sugar of a person practicing intermittent fasting reduced 3–6% while their insulin reduced by 20–31%. You can find this study here.

Reduced Oxidative Stress

Oxidative stress normally happens when your body has a higher production of free radicals than normal: free radicals include reactive oxygen species. These unstable molecules are normally caused by poorly functioning mitochondria. Such molecules carry reactive electrons, which either take an electron or give up an electron when they encounter other molecules.

When that happens, the result is usually a fast chain reaction from one molecule to the other. That then ends up creating more of these free radicals that causes the connections between atoms in the DNA, cellular membrane, and the essential proteins to break apart and destroy. These damages not only stress your body out but also age you since your cells are constantly being damaged.

What intermittent fasting does is that it lowers your blood sugar levels, which automatically forces your cells to turn to a survival process. When this happens, the cells quickly remove any mitochondria that are unhealthy and substitute them with new ones that are healthy as time goes on. This activity is the one that reduces the production of free radicals, which translates to a reduction in oxidative stress.

Reduced Risk of Cancer

The relationship between intermittent fasting and cancer has been heavily debated upon up to date. Some people suggest that intermittent fasting reduces the risk of cancer while others believe that more research needs to be done. But if this research is anything to go by, then intermittent fasting can really help you reduce the risk of cancer.

The study consisted of 10 cancer patients. Half of them were subjected to intermittent fasting before going for a chemotherapy session while the other half were not. After the two groups went for chemotherapy, it was discovered that the cancer patients who practiced intermittent fasting experienced reduced side effects and even had better cure rates than their counterparts did.

Cancer is usually caused by uncontrolled growth of cells, which mainly depend on the energy that comes from glucose to grow. Therefore, when you fast, you cut the energy channel that the cells need to grow. This causes the abnormal cells to stop growing completely or slow down.

Longevity

One of the most sort-after benefits of intermittent fasting is its ability to help you live a longer life. Numerous studies in rats have proven that intermittent fasting can actually extend your life span. In one of the rat studies, it was seen that rats that fasted daily lived 83% longer than those ones that didn't fast. Check out the study in the site below.

Now that you know how you can benefit from intermittent fasting, the next step is for you to find out how you can start practicing intermittent fasting and the methods that you will be using. The chapter below has all that information and more so read on.

Five Effective Ways to Lose Weight

Practicing intermittent fasting is just a simple process. It only needs you to be attentive to detail to succeed. The amazing thing about intermittent fasting is that there are various intermittent fasting methods you can choose. In this book, we will highlight five effective intermittent fasting methods that you can adopt and lose weight. Once you learn about the five methods, you can choose the most suitable one.

1. The 5:2 Diet

The 5:2 pattern of eating was originally popularized by Michael Mosley who was a doctor and a journalist.

Basically, the 5:2 diet is a way of eating that involves 5 days of regular eating in a week and then lowering calorie intake for the remaining 2 days of the week.

How to do it

The first thing that you need to do is to come up with a timetable that indicates when you eat normally and the days you restrict your calorie intake.

When making the timetable you should make sure that the two fasting days don't follow each other because if they do, you may end up straining your body and making this diet harder than it should be. Below is a simple example of a timetable that you can use.

DAYS	THE FAST DIET
MONDAY	FASTING
TUESDAY	FREE DAY
WEDNESDAY	FREE DAY
THURSDAY	FASTING
FRIDAY	FREE DAY
SATURDAY	FREE DAY
SUNDAY	FREE DAY

The five days that have been labeled free days are the days that you will be eating normally. With that being said, it is important to understand that eating normally does not mean you binge on processed food (binging won't enable you to lose weight and enjoy the benefits of intermittent fasting). It only means that you should eat the same amount of food that you usually eat: around 2000 calories for women and 2500 calories for men.

On those 2 days that you have marked fasting, you will be eating a quarter of your daily meal. If you are a woman, you will be consuming only 500 calories per day, and if you are a man, you will be required to consume 600 calories per day. On those days that you restrict your calorie intake, divide your calories into two meals, 300 calories per meal for the men and 250 calories for the women.

If you want to make your fasting day less dreadful, you can try finding foods that are low in calorie but fill you up faster. Such foods include broth-based soups, watermelon, green smoothies made of spinach, mustard, collards, kales, lentils, broccoli, celery, zucchini, and many others. It is also advisable to take a lot of water in your 2 days of fasting. This is because when you are hydrated, water eliminates the false feelings of hunger and that helps in reducing your appetite.

Who should NOT do the 5:2 diet?

This intermittent fasting method is very beneficial, but it is not for everyone. For instance, you should not get started on this diet for the following reasons:

- You are trying to conceive

- You are breastfeeding

- You are sensitive to blood sugar levels

- You have a history of eating disorders

2. Eat-Stop-Eat

This is another amazing type of intermittent fasting that gives you a different angle of fasting than the 5:2 diet. The eat-stop-eat method was discovered and made popular by Brad Pilon who had a background in the sports supplement industry and nutrition. Pilon based this method on the fact that brief and regular fasts eventually end up promoting weight loss and retention of muscles better than diets, which eliminate specific foods.

Basically, eat-stop-eat is a method that involves 24-hour fasting for once or twice in a week and then eating normally on the remaining days.

How to do it

As you have seen above, eat-stop-eat is a simple method that only requires you to take a complete 24 hours break from food. When starting this method, the first thing that you are supposed to do is to come up with the actual day for fasting. As a beginner, it's easier for you to start with 1 day fasting per week and then graduating to 2 days of fasting per week once you get used to fasting.

Many people perceive eat-stop-eat to be a difficult method, but it is really not. It's usually as simple as fasting from Monday 8 p.m. after taking your supper until Tuesday at 8 p.m. The only two meals that you will have to skip in this method are your breakfast and lunch. The best time to start fasting is after you have taken your dinner. This is because you will spend 8–

10 hours of your fasting time sleeping, which will be less stressful for you.

During fasting, do not eat anything except zero-calorie beverages. Some of the beverages that you can drink include water, coffee, tea, and diet soda. When taking tea and coffee, avoid milk and sugar because they are high in calories and can affect the benefits that you are supposed to get from the fast.

What is the best time for you to fast?

The best time to fast is when you are busy. If you know you will have a busy day at the office, you can start your fast the previous day at 8p.m. so that your fast falls on a busy day, which will leave you with little to no time to think about eating.

You can also schedule your fast to fall on a dinner or on a party. For instance, if you have been invited for a party on a Saturday evening, you can start fasting on Friday 8p.m so that you can break your fast at the party where you will get to eat all you want without feeling guilty. However, don't binge.

On your five free days, you can eat anything you want so long as it's in moderation. You should avoid overeating or eating too much junk food because it may slow down your progress. The best thing for you to do is to just eat normal as if you have not fasted.

But what happens if you cannot fast for 24 hours?

If for some reason you cannot fast for 24 hours, there is still hope for you because there is another approach you can use. That approach is called taking it slow.

Here is how to execute it. Test the waters by fasting and find out how long you can go without eating. If you managed to go for only 15 hours, try to add an hour in your next fast, which will be the following week. Gradually add the hours until you reach a point where you can fast for a whole 24 hours and then start working on how to do 2 fasts in a week.

How can you boost your weight loss?

In order to lose more weight, you can do exercises like weight training on the days that you are not fasting. This will also help you build and maintain your muscles. Below is a training schedule that you can follow to help with your effort to lose weight.

Day 1

- Do two sets of leg extensions for 10 reps.

- Do two sets for dumbbell lunges for 10 reps per foot.

- Do two sets of seated calf raises for 10 reps.

Day 2

- Do two sets of seated cable rows for 10 reps.

- Do two sets of pull-ups for 10 reps.

- Do two sets of one arm dumbbell preacher curl for 10 reps.

Day 3

- Do two sets of barbell bench press-wide grip of 10 reps.

- Do two sets of push-ups with feet elevated for 10 reps.

- Do two sets of front dumbbell raises for 10 reps.

Engaging in the above exercises will burn more calories leading to weight loss and building muscles.

3. The Warrior Diet

The warrior diet was discovered by Ori Hofmekler who was a fitness expert. The diet involves fasting for 20 hours and feasting at night within a window of 4 hours.

This method is called the warrior diet because when Hofmekler came up with this method, he got his inspiration from looking at warrior societies like Rome and ancient Sparta and studying how they used to function. He noticed that the warrior society consisted of lean and muscular people and then discovered that they were lean because they ate little food during the day and feasted on their hunt during the night.

Basically, the idea behind the warrior diet is mainly under eating during the day and overeating during the night. That is why you can eat small portions of food during the 20 hours of fasting because the idea is not to starve you. Your focus in this method should be to keep it simple by just eating like an ancient warrior.

How to do it

The warrior diet is very different from the three-meals-per-day diet that you are always used to. For this reason, it is not advisable to adopt the diet and move right into fasting for 20 hours a day immediately.

It is much better to take baby steps in your journey to fasting for 20 hours. If you don't, you might experience unpleasant side effects like light-headedness and weakness that will make you want to quit. Therefore, the best thing for you to do is to ease into the warrior diet. How can you do that?

Start by gradually adding some short periods of controlled fasting for a couple of days per week. For example, you can start by skipping breakfast twice in a week then eating regularly for the rest of the week. Skip two more breakfast in the following week. Now move to skipping lunch and repeat the gradual process until you reach a point where you are fasting for 20 hours and only feasting at night.

The good thing about the warrior diet is that it actually allows you to eat small portions of whole and raw foods like vegetables and fruits, small servings of proteins, and beverages like water, tea, and coffee. The small meals give your body that extra energy that it needs to keep on going during the fast, which is a huge advantage for you.

Once you are through with the 20 hours fast, you can have a huge meal anytime within the 4 hours window. Break your fast first with some broths, then take vegetables and meat or seafood, and if you are still hungry, you can eat some carbohydrates.

Exercises

The warrior diet is not just about fasting during the day and feasting during the night. It also involves some little exercising during the day when you are fasting.

Ancient warriors used to work or hunt during the daytime. Therefore, in order to adopt their lifestyle fully, you will need to do some exercises during the day. Some of these exercises include strength training exercises like high jumps, squats, pull-ups, and press-ups and high-intensity cardio activity like frog jumps and sprints.

The best way you can execute these exercises is by setting aside 30 minutes every day where you can do three different exercises two sets of 5 minutes each. Before the exercise, you can take a glass of protein shake that will go a long way in keeping you energized.

If you can adapt to this method fully, your body will turn into a fat burning machine, and that will help you in your weight loss and muscle gain goals.

4. Alternate Day Fasting

The alternate day fasting, which is also known as fasting every other day, is a unique and easy to follow method of intermittent fasting. This is because it gives you the opportunity to eat moderately instead of doing a full fast.

This method was initially formulated by James Johnson M.D. who designed it for disciplined dieters who have a specific weight goal. Since then, it has grown in popularity especially with people who love having a cheat day on their diet.

The concept behind alternate day fasting is pretty simple. Eat a limited amount of food on one day and then eat normal on the next day. For example, you can eat a small amount of food on Monday and then follow that up by eating normally on Tuesday. You should then spread out this pattern of eating throughout the week to have 3 days of limited food intake and 4 days of eating normally.

How to do it

As you have seen above, this method requires fasting every other day, so the first step that you should take when starting is come up with a timetable that will show you when you are supposed to fast and when you are supposed to eat normally. Below is a good example of an eating timetable.

DAYS	DIET
MONDAY	FAST
TUESDAY	FREE DAY
WEDNESDAY	FAST
THURSDAY	FREE DAY
FRIDAY	FAST
SATURDAY	FREE DAY
SUNDAY	FREE DAY

On your fasting day/down day, eat less food than you actually eat on your normal days. But what amount are we talking about? The amount that you are supposed to eat should be one-fifth of what you eat on a normal day.

Let's assume that you take 2000 calories if you are a woman or 2500 calories if you are a man during your normal day of eating. In your low-calorie day, divide 2000 calories for the woman and 2500 calories for the men by one-fifth to get 400 and 500 calories, respectively. This means that, on your low-calorie day, you will take in 400 calories if you are a woman and 500 calories if you are a man.

When it comes to eating and drinking on your down day, there are no general rules of how you can go about it. Some people fancy eating one big meal in the morning while others divide their limited calories into two to three meals in a day.

The best way to make your low-calorie days easier is by taking replacement shakes. Replacement shakes are usually very filling and low in calories. The second way to make your down day less stressful is by focusing on eating nutritious high-protein foods and vegetables, which will feel you up faster without having to eat too much calories. Below are some of the foods that will feel up faster.

- Soups: soups usually make you fuller than if you were to take the soup's ingredients on their own. Vegetable soups are the best, and you can take them with a fruit.

- Salad with lean meat

- Lean meat with vegetables

- Yogurt with berries

- Eggs and vegetables

The above foods are all safe to eat as long as they don't exceed 500 calories for men and 400 for woman.

If your main goal for intermittent fasting is weight loss, you are going to love alternate day fasting. This is because it works so perfectly when it comes to weight loss. The reason behind that is the way you mix a fasting day with a cheat day. How is that beneficial? You may wonder. It's simple, when you go for long periods of time without eating, your leptin levels drop, which automatically slows down your rate of fat loss.

However, because this method has a cheat day, your leptin levels rise up again and increase the rate of fat loss when you eat. Therefore, this method through a cheat day prevents you from stagnated fat loss.

5. The 16/8 Method

The 16/8 method which is also known as Leangains was discovered by Martin Berkhan who was a nutritional expert and a personal trainer. This method was designed mostly for people who like building muscles with minimum fat accumulation.

The idea behind 16/8 method is usually very simple: fast for 16 hours every day and only eat within a window of 8 hours. If you are a man, you can handle the 16/8 time frame, but if you are a woman, it will be more natural for you to fast for 14 hours in a day and restrict your daily eating window to 10 hours a day.

How to do it

The 16/8 method is usually as easy as deciding not to eat anything after dinner, then skipping your next day's breakfast and eating your next meal at lunch time.

There are so many ways you can implement the 16/8 method, but the best way is by starting the fast at 7 p.m. or 8 p.m. when you are through with your dinner. This is the best way because you will get to spend 10 hours out of 16 hours of fasting while sleeping.

That means that the hours of consciously fasting will be reduced to 6 hours, which will automatically make your fasting less stressful.

During the fast, do not eat any calories. However, since it can be hard for you to go a whole 16 hours without consuming anything, this method allows you to take some beverages. These beverages include the following:

- Water: Drinking water normally helps you suppress your hunger and adding cinnamon or lemon helps you to suppress your hunger even more.

- Coffee and tea: These two beverages are so important to your body because they do not just suppress your hunger but they also increase the fat burning intensity of intermittent fasting. Talk of killing two birds with one stone!

- Green tea: Green tea has various active bioactive properties like EGCG and caffeine that can aid in weight loss by boosting metabolism. The various bioactive agents also have the ability to interact with various hormones that trigger the breakdown of fat.

The 16/8 method as you saw above was also designed with fitness in mind. So how can you schedule your workouts around this method? If you like working out in the morning, then you will have no choice but to work out on an empty stomach.

Of course, it won't be easy and that's why I am going to give you a secret that you can use to make your workouts less stressful. The secret is for you to take a BCAA protein shake before starting your morning workout be it being jogging; calisthenic exercises like pull-ups, sit-ups, and press-ups; or weightlifting exercises.

Just take a 10-gram powdered BCAA. Mix it with water to make a protein shake and then follow the schedule below:

- 6 a.m.: Use 5–15 minutes taking 10 grams of protein shake

- 6–7 a.m.: Exercise

- 8 a.m.: Take 10 grams of protein shake

- 10 a.m.: Take 10 grams of protein shake

Once you break your fast, avoid overeating and eating junk food because they will interfere with your weight loss efforts. You can have two to three meals during your eating window comprising of whole unprocessed foods like seafood, fish, lean meat, and eggs; fresh fruits like watermelon, mangoes, avocado, and bananas; and vegetables like kales, celery, and broccoli.

Tip: If you like to work out in the evening, you can schedule your workouts 1–2 hours after you've taken your first meal while following the 16/8 method (assuming you fast overnight from around 7–9 up to around 11.a.m.–1 p.m.).

Those are the five effective methods of intermittent fasting that you can use to lose weight and build lean muscles.

The Scientific Approach to Intermittent Fasting

What does the general medical community think about intermittent fasting?

Many diets originate from legitimate scientific studies but are often altered by the time the diets reach the masses. This is because to market the diets, the benefits of the diets are often exaggerated and the risks are played down. The science behind the diets takes a back seat to marketing.

With this being the way things are, health professionals automatically dismiss all diets that come along as just another fad diet with questionable health benefits. What is good about the diets that come along is thrown out along with the bad, and in their eyes, intermittent fasting is no different.

Medical professionals fear that intermittent fasting encourages binge eating of junk food since this practice does not concern itself with caloric restriction when it is time to eat.

However, the medical community in general has more interest in making money off of obese and sick people than it has in educating people on ways they can reverse and/or prevent diseases through natural means.

What do the proponents of intermittent fasting say about this practice?

Mild versions of the intermittent fasting only require 14 to 16 hours without food, while more extreme versions include days at a time without food.

People who favor intermittent fasting argue that healthy food and a variety of food is what they encourage whenever fasters eat.

Enthusiasts say that intermittent fasting is a healthy lifestyle as nature intended for man, keeping extra weight off while significantly reducing risk factors for disease, increasing one's lifespan, and giving the people who adopt this practice an appearance of youthfulness. Therefore, proponents of intermittent fasting do not view it as just a fad diet.

After eating the healthy food that the body wants for a while, the body increasingly desires more of the quality food and no longer wants junk food. In some cases, the junk food is no longer even tolerated.

The Scientific Research

Calorie restriction is undernourishment without malnourishment. In other words, calorie restriction means one eats fewer calories than they did before without losing nourishment. The effects restriction calorie intake on the health of both humans and animals have been conducted in many studies, but the effects of intermittent fasting on humans has not been clinically studied in mass.

The health effects of intermittent fasting are similar to those of calorie restriction (low-calorie) diets. The mild level of stress put onto the cells by both calorie restriction and intermittent fasting bring about resistance to both environmental and metabolic stress without doing harm.

Studies of the effects of intermittent fasting on animals proved that this practice is good for them. According to Mark Mattson, who is the senior investigator for the National Institute on Aging (a US National Institutes of Health division), in many studies, intermittent fasting showed improvement in diseases, reduced oxidative stress, and preserved memory and learning function in the animals studied.

What have clinical studies on humans proven concerning intermittent fasting?

Though widespread clinical studies of the effects of intermittent fasting on humans have not yet taken, Mattson participated in several studies of humans where intermittent fasting was combined with restricted calorie intake.

Mattson found during the course of these studies that the body goes to the fat stores for energy after 10–16 hours of fasting. In addition to significant weight loss of stubborn pounds, many health issues proved to be drastically corrected by this combination of intermittent fasting and low-calorie intake of healthy, quality food.

Mattson theorized that the reason for the body's capability to deal with stress and combat disease is that fasting puts cells under mild stress, which makes the cells adapt to the stress. He stated, "There is considerable similarity between how cells respond to the stress of exercise and how cells respond to intermittent fasting."

Ancient man hunted during times when they hadn't eaten for several hours. Thus, exercising during the end of their daily mini fasts caused optimum burning of fat because their bodies were already burning fat for energy at that stage.

When they did eat, the food they ate was fresh meat, fish, plants, fruit, and nuts, which are the types of healthy food people eat on the intermittent fasting diets when proper use of the diet is being practiced.

What studies have been done on the effects of calorie restriction on the human heart?

As previously stated, extensive studies on how restricting calories affects humans have been conducted. Intense studies on how calorie restriction affects humans with heart disease in particular have been conducted, and the results were very positive.

One study indicated that a calorie-restricted diet significantly improved the average blood pressure, fasting insulin, carotid IMT, fasting glucose, body mass index, C-reactive protein, body fat percentage, and platelet-derived growth factor AB in human study subjects.

What are the metabolic effects of intermittent fasting?

Intermittent fasting causes the body to respond in several ways, but the exact reasons for the responses are not fully understood. The following is what the studies have shown:

Stress responses: Short-term fasting creates mild stress on the body. The body responds by compensating in the areas of glucose-related protein, corticosterone and glucocorticoid receptors.

Neuroprotection: The body responds to short-term fasting by upregulating neurotropic factors to assure survival of neurons and to make new connections. Chaperone proteins are upregulated as well, which as a result protect cells from damaging and dying.

Cytoprotective activity (as relates to seizures and epilepsy): Intermittent fasting proved to have better efficiency than calorie restriction in the ketogenic metabolic pathway. Twice as much ketone forms in intermittent fasting than in calorie restriction. In a study, increased ketone shows neuroprotectivity for sufferers of Parkinson's and Alzheimer's diseases.

Improvements related to insulin and glucose: Since short-term fasting limits the availability of glucose, the body finds alternative sources of energy. One of these sources is a fatty acid-based metabolism. Long-term availability of glucose leads to protein damage, which proves that intermittent fasting does a body good.

In addition to non-enzymatic glycation, calorie restriction prevents oxyradical damage and production.

Calorie restriction and intermittent fasting both reduce insulin and glucose levels, but for serum IGF-1 and serum beta-hydroxybutyrate levels, they have different effects. Intermittent fasting elevates both serum IGF-1 and serum beta-hydroxybutyrate levels. The IGF-1 levels are increased because of the increased production of growth hormone.

Both calorie restriction and intermittent fasting increases insulin sensitivity in monkeys.

Mediation of cytokines: Interferon-gamma (IFN-g) enhances synaptogenesis, controls neurogenesis, and regulates synaptic plasticity.

Intermittent fasting elevates IFN-g in the hippocampus, which protects it against excitotoxicity. Calorie restriction does the same thing in circulating leukocytes.

In animals, tumor necrosis factor a (TNF-a) triggers resistance to insulin, which causes problems due to increased glucose levels in aged animals.

Both intermittent fasting and calorie restriction results to a decrease of adipose tissue, leading to a reduction of TNF-a secretion. Nuclear factor kappa-light-chain-enhancer of activated B cells (NF-kB) also reduces TNF-a secretion. Both intermittent fasting and calorie restriction upregulate NF-kB.

Leptin and adiponectin: Adipose tissue secretes adiponectin and leptin, which suppress appetite. It is theorized that leptin deregulates the thyroid hormones in calorie restriction functions.

Calorie restriction elevates adiponectin by upregulating AMP-regulated protein kinase. Adiponectin triggers sensitivity to insulin. Also, protein kinase protects neurons from stress due to metabolic causes.

Sirtuins: Silent information regulator gene 2 (SIR2), when upregulated, can increase a person's lifespan, and it decreases one's life when it is downregulated.

SIR1 is the mammalian analog. It affects both health and longevity through the following: (1) the regulation of adiponectin gene expression, (2) glucose homeostasis gluconeogenesis, (3) attenuates adipogenesis increased fat metabolism and mobilization, and (4) modulates inflammatory response.

Both intermittent fasting and calorie restriction increase SIR1 protein secretion.

SIR expressions are upregulated by cell stressors. This leads to the assumption that SIR genes could be activated by intermittent fasting and calorie restriction through that process as well through their mild stress inducing capacity.

Peroxisome proliferator-activated receptor (PPAR): Gene expression is regulated by PPAR. In mammals, IPGC-1 (its gamma coactivator 1) is regulated closely through diet restriction. Calorie restriction remedies the age-dependent decrease of PGC-1, which makes it likely that it increases lifespan.

FoxO transcription factors: FoxO proteins regulate genes. They regulate the expression of energy metabolism-related proteins. Glucose metabolism, DNA repair, cell death through Fas ligand, reactive oxygen species detoxification are all examples of FoxO function.

Myths About Intermittent Fasting

There are a few myths about intermittent fasting that need to be addressed. Some of the top ones are as follows:

Myth 1: Intermittent fasting is starving the body.

Fasting gives the body rest and the opportunity to bring optimal health to the body. This is how man was designed to eat, and it is how our much-healthier ancestors ate. When we break our fast, we eat healthy. Therefore, there is no malnourishment.

Myth 2: We should eat every two or so hours.

No. You were not designed to eat three square meals per day, as modern society teaches us. Your body needs the opportunity to heal itself instead of constantly digesting food.

Myth 3: Breakfast is the most important meal of the day.

Technically, breakfast is whenever you are breaking your fast, not an assigned time of day. Additionally, it is important for all meals to be healthy.

Myth 4: Intermittent fasting would make you tired.

No. It actually gives you energy because your body is not having to expend 70% of its energy to digesting food constantly.

Myth 5: Intermittent fasting would make your muscles waste away.

Not true, especially if you include lots of protein in your food choices.

Myth 6: Intermittent fasting would mess up my metabolism.

Intermittent fasting actually boosts metabolism by eliminating wastes and toxins, activating human growth hormone, regulating digestion, training the body to burn fat, regulating blood sugar, improving eating habits, and slowing aging.

Myth 7: Intermittent fasting is hard to do.

It is not hard to do, especially if the method you choose involves just a daily mini fast. The method you choose depends on your goals, and some methods are harder than others. No matter which method you choose, it is advisable to have healthy food on hand when you break your fast so that you wouldn't be tempted to go through a drive-thru for unhealthy food. Pre-prepped recipe ingredients for recipes would also help.

Myth 8: Intermittent fasting is unhealthy.

It is the opposite. The healthiest people in the world barely eat. Your body needs the opportunity to rest and to heal itself instead of constantly digesting food. Bodybuilders fast regularly to improve their health.

What You Need to Know About Hunger

We are all familiar with the rumblings of our tummies when we are hungry. The thought of intermittently fasting or restricting calories therefore might not be a comforting one.

When we realize that intermittent fasting and/or restricting calories is actually a very healthy practice that can make us feel and look really good, sleep better, think better, perform at work better, and have more energy, we can begin to embrace the notion. We can then figure out which method fits our goals and how to best fit intermittent fasting and/or calorie restriction into our life, and we can learn tricks to keep from feeling hungry.

It is encouraging to consider that intermittent fasting manages our appetites by controlling hunger hormones through the production of a hormone called leptin. Leptin is secreted after the body starts to burn the stored fat for energy and tells the brain to shut off the hunger hormone, ghrelin.

Also noteworthy is the fact that sometimes we are thirsty rather than hungry. Even if that isn't the case, drinking water, tea, or coffee (without cream or sugar) or eating food with a high amount of liquid in them can take the edge off.

The number one way to prevent ourselves from feeling the most intense hunger, however, is to *omit carbohydrates and sugar from the diet* because intense hunger pangs are often caused by wide fluctuations in blood sugar.

High amounts of carbs and sugar cause high amounts of insulin to be made, which causes the sugar to be utilized for energy. The unused food is stored as fat, and a sudden drop in the blood sugar level follows, making us feel really hungry. Omitting most of the carbs or sugars we eat would therefore go a long way toward helping us to not ever feel famished.

Candida overgrowth and parasite infestation

Of course, if a person has *candida overgrowth* or *parasite infestation* throughout their digestive system, this is easier said than done because *both of these conditions make us crave a lot of sugar.* That is because these creatures require sugar to live. Sugar is highly addictive without the added craving for it that candida and parasites bring on.

If you have food allergies and think you have candida, you'll benefit from using an allergy specialist to address both the food allergies and candida overgrowth.

Symptoms of candida include the following:

- Food allergies or sensitivities
- A creamy whitish discharge that comes from lesions or your tongue,
  tonsils, roof of your mouth, or inner cheeks
- Red or purple spots on skin similar to eczema
- Itching in personal areas
- Cracking around the mouth or an infected area
- Swelling in the mouth, sex organs, skin, or intestines
- Much discomfort when advanced
- Irritable bowel disease
- Fatigue
- Mood disorders.

If you have a distended abdomen and can't figure out why, you might have parasite infestation.

Symptoms of parasite infestation include the following:

- Abdominal distension
- Diarrhea
- Mucous in stools
- Smelly stools
- Cramps and gas
- Coughing
- Fever
- Vomiting
- General weakness.

With either condition, you would decrease hunger and make huge initial progress in both girth and health by flushing the digestive tract through frequent colonics or enemas at home.

The next step would be to starve and weaken the hangers-on by depriving them of all forms of sugar. Then, you would flush the dead candida and/or worms out.

If you are under a doctor's care for candida, you would also actively kill the fungus by taking the prescribed Nystatin or something similar. He would also have you add probiotics and cold-pressed flaxseed oil to your diet.

If eating healthy is a drastic change from what you normally eat, you will feel worse before you feel better, having headaches and a strong urge to eat sugary or starchy foods. That is because the detoxification process makes a traffic jam out in the bloodstream. Flushing much of it out through colonics or enemas would help to lessen this effect and speed up the process of elimination.

You would do well to rid yourself of candida and/or parasites at the same time that you adopt your new eating lifestyle since treating candida and parasites involve a strict diet anyway.

Once your digestive tract is clean, your body will be able to absorb nutrients much more efficiently. Your body will only want quality food. It will also want less food, including sweets, naturally.

Frequently Asked Questions

Question Isn't intermittent fasting actually starvation?

Answer No, especially if only quality food is eaten when it is time to eat. Fasting gives the body rest and the opportunity to bring optimal health to the body. This is how man was designed to eat, and it is how our much-healthier ancestors ate.

Question Shouldn't I eat every two or so hours?

Answer No. You were not designed to eat three square meals per day, as modern society teaches us. Your body needs the opportunity to heal itself instead of constantly digesting food.

Question Isn't breakfast the most important meal of the day?

Answer Technically, breakfast is whenever you are breaking your fast, not an assigned time of day. Additionally, it is important for all meals to be healthy.

Question Wouldn't intermittent fasting make me tired?

Answer No. It actually gives you energy because your body is not having to expend 70% of its energy to digesting food constantly.

Question Wouldn't intermittent fasting make my muscles waste away?

Answer No, especially if you include lots of protein in your food choices.

Question Wouldn't intermittent fasting mess up my metabolism?

Answer No. Intermittent fasting boosts metabolism by eliminating wastes and toxins, activating human growth hormone, regulating digestion, training the body to burn fat, regulating blood sugar, improving eating habits, and slowing aging.

Question Isn't intermittent fasting hard to do?

Answer No, especially if the method you choose involves just a daily mini fast. The method you choose depends on your goals, and some methods are harder than others. No matter which method you choose, it is advisable to have healthy food on hand for when you break your fast so that you wouldn't be tempted to go through a drive-thru for unhealthy food. Pre-prepped recipe ingredients for recipes would also help.

Question Isn't intermittent fasting unhealthy?

Answer No. It is the opposite. The healthiest people in the world barely eat. Your body needs the opportunity to rest and to heal itself instead of constantly digesting food.

Question If I lose weight by fasting intermittently, I still wouldn't look good if I don't also work out, right?

Answer The weight would drop off, but exercise always helps to tone the body!

Question What are the health benefits of intermittent fasting besides weight loss?

Answer Fasting clears the head, preserves memory, and aids in learning. It retards the aging process through the increase in HGH, mitochondria energy, and the reduction in stress. It burns fat and helps to make you feel "clean" inside, decreases food cravings for bad foods, and increases desire for quality foods. Fasting aids in the production of testosterone and improves the sex drive. It helps you to sleep. It also increases insulin sensitivity, thus making strides in the fight against Type-II Diabetes. Through Fasting, the risk of breast cancer is reduced, as well as the risk of heart disease. It also reduces blood pressure. Fasting reduces LDL and overall cholesterol levels and improves pancreatic function. All of these benefits come from just NOT eating for a few extra hours!

Question Why use intermittent fasting?

Answer In addition to quickly losing weight, intermittent fasting facilitates better detoxification, manages hunger while losing weight, creates health, and promotes longevity.

Question Which fasting method allows me to retain muscle the best?

Answer The Eat-Stop-Eat method.

Question What is a good vegetable shake for use on low-calorie days?

Answer A smoothie made of spinach, mustard greens, collards, kales, lentils, broccoli, celery, and zucchini is one example.

Question Should I eat what is normal for me or should I eat extra healthy when eating on an intermittent fast diet?

Answer If you are only eating junk food, you need to upgrade the quality of the food you eat on a normal basis. Quality food would speed up the process of losing weight and would also greatly improve your overall health and appearance. One other key factor is to not binge eat unless you are on the warrior diet and eating quality food.

Question Besides eating quality food, how can I speed up the process of losing weight?

Answer Exercise toward the end of your fasting time, which is when the body is burning fat instead of food or glycogen.

Question What foods would fill me up faster than others on low-calorie days?

Answer Vegetable shakes, vegetable soups and fruit, salad with lean meat, lean meat with vegetables, yogurt with berries, and eggs and vegetables. Healthy oils.

Question Which is the best intermittent fasting method if the goal is mainly weight loss?

Answer Alternate day fasting

Question I want to conceive a baby. Which method should I *avoid*?

Answer The 5:2 Diet.

Question I am breast feeding. Which method should I *avoid*?

Answer The 5:2 Diet.

Question I am sensitive to low blood sugar levels. Which method should I *avoid*?

Answer The 5:2 Diet.

Question I have a history of eating disorders. Which method should I *avoid*?

Answer The 5:2 Diet.

Question I want to lose weight but not my muscles. Which method should I use?

Answer The Eat-Stop-Eat Diet.

Question I want to be lean and muscular, and I'm willing to work out to maintain being lean and muscular. Which method should I use?

Answer The Warrior Diet.

Question Which method is the easiest one to follow?

Answer The Alternate Day Fasting Diet would be just about the easiest because you eat every day. It's just that 3 days a week you limit the number of calories you take in.

Question How can I make my low-calorie days easier?

Answer Vegetable shakes, vegetable soups and fruit, salad with lean meat, lean meat with vegetables, yogurt with berries, and eggs and vegetables.

Question What method allows me to cheat?

Answer The Alternate Day Fasting Diet. That is because you will be eating few calories on the next day, most of the time.

Question How many calories do I eat on "low-calorie days?"

Answer Eat 20% of whatever your normal level of intake is, which would likely be about 500 calories for men and 400 for women.

The Action Plan

1. Decide what your goal is. Do you just want to lose weight? Do you want to gain muscle? Do you have situations in your life such as breast feeding that require a method that will not interfere? Have your goal in mind when you go to choose the method you want.

2. Select the fasting plan that fits your goals. If you have done step one, just read through the fasting methods. One of them will stand out to you. Consult your physician if you are taking meds and think you need your proposed plan cleared with him. You'll likely eventually get off of the meds.

3. Decide how you can fit the chosen method you choose into your life. One common way to fit the fasting lifestyle into one's life is to start the fast after dinner on certain days and then exercise in the morning, and so on.

4. Write out a menu for the week, along with a shopping list. You will want to be prepared to get everything you will need for your future success! If you are addressing candida, parasites, or leaky gut at the same time as you are addressing weight loss and general health, you'll need to make sure you only shop for and eat the foods you can have.

5. Purchase what you'll need. If you plan to lift weights and don't have weights, obviously now is the time to buy some. Will you start utilizing a dehydrator for the kinds of food you will eat? Do you have the food ingredients that you'll need? Buy what you need.

6. Pre-prep food. If you need to have some pre-prepped food items on hand, ready to go when you come off of your fast and need to quickly prepare yourself a healthy dish, you'll need to make them.

7. Get started! You might have your last meal of junk food and then start your fast.

Hey! Are you enjoying this book and are you receiving value from it? I would really appreciate if you could leave a review on amazon.

Click here to leave a review on Amazon!

(If you read this on an iOS device please 'swipe' to the left at the end of the book to leave a review.)

Twenty Super Healthy, Healing Recipes

Main Dish Recipes

Coconut Curried Chicken

This recipe makes 1–2 servings and takes about 45 minutes of preparation.

What's in It

- Sea salt (to taste)
- Cinnamon (1 teaspoon)
- Ginger (1 teaspoon)
- Garlic (4 cloves)
- Curry powder (2 tablespoons)
- White onion (1 onion)
- Water chestnuts (1 cup)
- Broccoli (2 cups)
- Coconut milk (1 14-ounce can)
- Chicken breasts (2 pounds)

How It's Made

- Mince the ginger. Set aside.
- Mince the garlic cloves. Set aside.
- Slice the onion. Set aside.
- Heat skillet to a medium temperature.
- Add the coconut milk, broccoli, onion and chicken
- Cook for 15 minutes.
- Add the sea salt, cinnamon, ginger, garlic, curry powder and the water chesnuts.
- Reduce to medium-low heat.
- Cook for another 15 minutes.

Almond Encrusted Salmon

This recipe makes 2–4 servings and takes about 20 minutes of preparation.

What's in It

- Fresh spinach (4 cups)
- Grapeseed oil (2 tablespoons)
- Wild caught salmon fillets (4 fillets)
- Lemon zest (1 tablespoon)
- Pepper and sea salt (1 teaspoon)
- Parsley (2 tablespoon)
- Almonds (0.5 cup)
- Lemon juice (to taste)

How It's Made

- Grate the lemon. Set aside.
- Grind the almonds into a powder using a food processor or coffee grinder. Set aside.
- Mix the sea salt, pepper, parsley, lemon zest, and almond together on a plate.
- Coat the almond mixture on both sides of the salmon fillets.
- In a large skillet, heat oil over medium heat.
- Put the fillets into the skillet and cook sides for 5 minutes each.
- Place fillets on plate over a bed of spinach leaves.
- Squeeze fresh lemon juice over the top.

Asian Beef Stir Fry

This recipe makes 1–2 servings and takes about 30 minutes of preparation.

What's in It

- Red bell pepper (1 pepper)
- Bragg's liquid aminos (3 tablespoons)
- Snow peas (8 ounces)
- Grass-fed beef round steak, cut into strips (1 pound)
- Garlic, fresh (1 tablespoon)
- Honey (1 tablespoon)
- Ginger root, fresh (1 tablespoon)
- Grapeseed oil (1 tablespoon)
- Rice wine vinegar (2 tablespoons)
- Brown rice (personal choice as to how much)

How It's Made

- Cook brown rice to serve the stir fry on.
- Mix together the honey, vinegar, and liquid aminos using a small bowl. Set sauce aside.
- Slice the red bell pepper. Set aside.
- Cut the steak into strips. Set aside.
- Mince the garlic. Set aside.
- Mince the ginger root. Set aside.
- In a large skillet, heat oil over medium heat.
- Put the ginger and garlic into the skillet and then stir fry for about 30 seconds.
- Put the steak into the skillet and then stir fry until evenly browned.

- Put the snow peas and red bell pepper into the skillet and then stir fry for 3 minutes.
- Pour the sauce into the mixture. Bring pan contents to a boil, stirring constantly.
- Lower heat. Simmer for a few more minutes.
- Serve over the brown rice.

Spicy Walnut Tacos

This recipe makes 1–2 servings and takes about 10 minutes of preparation.

What's in It

- Cayenne pepper (1 pinch)
- Bragg's liquid aminos (2 teaspoons)
- Coriander (0.75 teaspoons)
- Ground cumin (1.5 teaspoons)
- Raw walnuts (1.5 cups)
- Lettuce (as desired)
- Salsa (to taste)
- Guacamole (to taste)

How It's Made

- Grind walnuts in food processor.
- Add the remaining ingredients and mix together in food processor.
- Serve in lettuce wraps with salsa and guacamole.

Cashew Chicken Lettuce Wraps

This recipe makes 1–2 servings and takes about 30 minutes of preparation.

What's in It

- Cashews (0.25 cup)
- Water chestnuts (1 8-ounce can)
- Bragg's liquid aminos (2 tablespoons)
- Scallions (1 bunch)
- Chicken breasts (1.5 pounds)
- Ginger root (1 tablespoon)
- Garlic (2 cloves)
- Honey (2 tablespoons)
- Pepper and sea salt (to taste)
- Grapeseed oil (2 tablespoons)

How It's Made

- Toast the cashews. Set aside.
- Drain and slice the water chestnuts. Set aside.
- Trim and slice the scallions. Set aside.
- Grate the ginger root. Set aside.
- Chop the garlic finely. Set aside.
- Cut the chicken breasts into 0.75-inch slices. Set aside.
- In a bowl, mix the Bragg's liquid aminos and honey. Set sauce aside.
- Heat the grapeseed oil in a large skillet over medium heat.
- Season the chicken strips with the sea salt and pepper.

- Cook the chicken, stir occasionally until it starts to turn brown, which is around 5 minutes.
- Add the garlic, ginger and scallions to the pan. Stir fry for 1 minute.
- Add the water chestnuts and sauce. Stir fry until chicken is cooked... about 4 minutes.
- Remove from heat.
- Spoon onto lettuce.
- Sprinkle with the toasted cashews.

Chicken Fajitas

This recipe makes 2 servings and takes about 45 minutes of preparation.

What's in It

- Spouted grain or brown rice tortillas (1 package)
- Organic black beans (1 can)
- Cumin (1 teaspoon)
- Chicken breast (2 pounds)
- Chili powder (1 teaspoon)
- Sea salt (1 teaspoon)
- Garlic (2 cloves)
- White onion (1 onion)
- Red bell pepper (1 pepper)
- Green bell pepper (1 pepper)
- Coconut oil (2 tablespoons)

How It's Made

- Chop the garlic cloves. Set aside.
- In a large skillet, heat oil over medium heat.
- Put the chicken into the skillet.
- Sprinkle with half of the garlic and half (0.5 teaspoon) of the sea salt.
- Cook until done.
- Remove from the heat. Let cool.
- Take the chicken out of the pan. Shred chicken apart with a knife and fork. Set aside.
- Add enough water to the skillet to cover the bottom.
- Add the onion, bell peppers, and the rest of the sea salt and garlic to the pan.

- Cook 5 – 10 minutes.
- Add the shredded chicken back to the pan.
- Season with chili powder and cumin.
- Cook until the vegetables are tender.
- Serve over tortillas. Top with black beans.

Chicken Basil Stir Fry

This recipe makes 2 servings and takes about 30 minutes of preparation.

What's in It

- Mirin (1 teaspoon, optional)
- Bragg's liquid aminos (2 teaspoons or to taste)
- Fresh basil (2 tablespoons)
- Chicken breast (1 pound)
- Carrots, small (2 carrots)
- Broccoli, small florets (2 cups)
- Orange peel (0.5 teaspoon)
- Shitake mushrooms (3 large mushrooms)
- Red onion, large (0.5 onion)
- Grapeseed oil (1 tablespoon)

How It's Made

- In a large skillet, heat oil over medium heat.
- Saute mushrooms, onions and orange peel until browned, about 3–5 minutes.
- Add carrots and broccoli to the skillet. Stir fry for 3–5 minutes. Place in bowl. Set aside.
- Replenish oil in the skillet if needed.
- Place chicken into the skillet. Cook for 5 minutes or until done.
- Put vegetables back into the skillet.
- Season with Bragg's liquid aminos, basil, and mirin.
- Cook 1 minute or until heated completely.

Bison Burgers

This recipe makes 2 servings and takes about 15 minutes of preparation.

What's in It

- Coconut oil (1 tablespoon)
- Black pepper and sea salt (to taste)
- Bragg's liquid aminos (1 teaspoon)
- Garlic powder (1 teaspoon)
- Onion powder (1 teaspoon)
- Cumin (1 teaspoon)
- Ground bison (2 pounds)

How It's Made

- In a large bowl, mix the meat with the cumin, onion powder, garlic powder, sea salt, and pepper.
- Form patties from the mixture.
- In a large skillet, heat oil over medium heat.
- Fry the patties. Flip once to cook the other side until they are done.
- Serve by itself or on a bed of greens.

Chicken Tenders

This recipe makes 2 servings and takes about 25 minutes of preparation.

What's in It

- Coconut oil (1 tablespoon)
- Brown rice flour or coconut flour (1 cup)
- Sea salt (to taste)
- Italian seasoning (to taste)
- Eggs (2 eggs)
- Chicken breasts (2 pounds)

How It's Made

- Cut the chicken breasts into strips. Set aside.
- In a bowl, beat the eggs. Add the sea salt and Italian seasoning to taste.
- Put the flour into a bowl or onto a plate.
- In the skillet, heat the coconut oil over medium heat.
- Dip the chicken strips into the beaten eggs and then roll strips in the flour.
- Fry the chicken strips, turning once, until fried to a golden brown color and done.

Bean Burgers

This recipe makes 2 servings and takes about 30 minutes of preparation.

What's in It

- Sea salt and black pepper (to taste)
- Lime juice (2 tablespoons)
- Cilantro, fresh (2 tablespoons)
- Tahini (2 tablespoons)
- Rosemary, fresh (1 tablespoon)
- Breadcrumbs, gluten free (0.5 cup)
- Coconut oil (2 tablespoons)
- Sweet onions (1.5 pounds)
- Garlic, fresh (6 cloves)
- Garbanzo beans, cooked (2 cups)
- Avacodo (1 avacado)
- Greens or sprouts (to taste)

How It's Made

- Mince the fresh rosemary, cilantro and garlic; slice the onions thinly. Set aside.
- Heat 1 tablespoon of the coconut oil in a large skillet.
- Saute onions until they are soft and start caramelizing. Then, season with sea pepper and salt.
- Put the seasoned onions into a bowl and then set aside.
- Blend garbanzo beans until smooth. Add to the bowl of onions.

- Add the lime juice, tahini, rosemary, cilantro, garlic and breadcrumbs to the bowl.
- Mix the contents of the bowl well and form into patties.
- Heat the remaining tablespoon of the coconut oil.
- Cook the burgers until they are done, flipping once.
- Serve with avocado slices and greens or sprouts.

Salad Recipes

Carrot Raisin Salad

This recipe makes 2 servings and takes about 10 minutes of preparation.

What's in It

- Peaches, frozen (1 cup)
- Stevia (0.25 teaspoon)
- Sea salt (0.5 teaspoon)
- Raisins (0.5 cup)
- Lemon juice (2 teaspoon)
- Homemade mayonnaise or Vegenaise with grapeseed oil (0.5 cup)
- Carrots (3 cups)

How It's Made

- Grate the carrots. Put into a bowl.
- Add the Stevia, sea salt, lemon juice, mayo/Vegenaise, raisins and carrots to the carrots.
- Refrigerate the mixture until ready to serve.
- Mix in frozen peaches when ready to serve.

Broccoli Salad

This recipe makes 2 servings and takes about 10 minutes of preparation.

What's in It

- Stevia (to taste)
- Red wine vinegar (2 tablespoons)
- Sunflower seeds (0.5 cup)
- Vegenaise with grapeseed oil or some other mayonnaise alternative (0.75 cup)
- Green onions (0.5 cup)
- Raisins (0.5 cup)
- Broccoli (1 bunch)

How It's Made

- Chop the broccoli.
- Chop the green onions.
- Mix all ingredients in a large bowl.
- Refrigerate.
- Serve cold.

Chicken Salad

This recipe makes 4 servings and takes about 10 minutes of preparation.

What's in It

- Sea salt (to taste)
- Walnuts (0.25 cup)
- Vegenaise with grapeseed oil or other mayonnaise alternative (0.7 cup)
- Lemon juice (2 teaspoons)
- Red grapes (1 cup)
- Celery (2–3 cups)
- Chicken, cooked (3–4 cups)

How It's Made

- Coarsely chop the celery and the walnuts (if not bought already chopped).
- Cut up pre-cooked chicken.
- Mix all ingredients together. Serve.

Side Dish Recipes

Grecian Spinach

This recipe makes 1–2 servings and takes about 20 minutes of preparation.

What's in It

- Feta cheese, crumbled (0.25 cup)
- Sea salt and pepper (to taste)
- Lemon peel (0.5 teaspoon)
- Baby spinach, fresh (16 ounces)
- Red onion (0.5 onion)
- Coconut oil (1 tablespoon)

How It's Made

- Cut up the onion into thin slices. Set aside.
- Wash and de-stem the spinach. Set aside.
- Grate the lemon peel. Set aside.
- In a large skillet, heat up the coconut oil over medium heat.
- Add the red onion to the skillet. Saute 2–3 minutes.
- Add the spinach to the skillet. Saute 2–3 minutes.
- Add the sea salt and pepper. Add the lemon peel. Stir in.
- Stir in the feta cheese just before serving.

Butternut Squash Casserole

This recipe makes 2 servings and takes about 1 hour of preparation.

What's in It

- Almonds, slivered (0.25 cup)
- Grade B maple syrup (2 tablespoons)
- Grapeseed oil (2 tablespoon)
- Unsweetened apple cider or juice (0.33 cup)
- Red onion, small (1 onion)
- Butternut squash, small (1 squash)

How It's Made

- Toast the almonds.
- Preheat oven to 350 degrees.
- Peel, halve, and de-seed squash. Cut into thin slices and place into 9 × 13 baking dish.
- Cut the onion into thin slices. Put into baking dish.
- Mix the grapeseed oil, syrup, and apple cider in a bowl. Pour over the squash and onions.
- Top with the toasted almonds.
- Cover the casserole with aluminum foil. Bake for 45 minutes or until tender.

Zucchini Skillet

This recipe makes 4 servings and takes about 30 minutes of preparation.

What's in It

- Black olives, ripe (2 tablespoons)
- Tomatoes, fresh (1 cup)
- Garlic powder (0.125 teaspoon)
- Sea salt (0.5 teaspoon)
- Basil, fresh (2 teaspoons)
- Zucchini (3 cups)
- Grapeseed oil (3 tablespoons)
- Onion (0.5 cup)

How It's Made

- Chop the onion. Put into a bowl. Set aside.
- Shred the zucchini coarsely. Put into the bowl with the onions. Set aside.
- Mince the basil. Put into the bowl with the onions and zucchini. Set aside.
- Dice the tomatoes. Set aside separately from the onion–zucchini–tomato mixture.
- Slice the olives. Set aside separately from the onion-zucchini-tomato mixture.
- In a large skillet, heat up the grapeseed oil over medium heat.
- Saute the zucchini, onions, basil, garlic powder and sea salt for 5–6 minutes.
- Put the tomatoes and olives on top.
- Cover. Cook for 5 more minutes.

Grainless Tabbouleh

This recipe makes 2 servings and takes about 30 minutes of preparation.

What's in It

- Black pepper, fresh (3 grinds)
- Sea salt (1 teaspoon)
- Lemon juice, fresh (2 tablespoons)
- Olive oil (2 tablespoons)
- Pine nuts (1 tablespoon)
- Mint leaves, fresh (1 cup)
- Celery (0.75 cup)
- Tomatoes (0.75 cup)
- Cucumbers, medium (2 cucumbers)
- Italian parsley (2 cups)
- Curly parsley (2 cups)

How It's Made

- Chop the mint leaves. Put into a bowl.
- Dice the celery. Add to the bowl with the mint leaves.
- Chop the tomatoes. Add to the bowl with the mint leaves and celery.
- Peel, de-seed and dice finely the cucumbers. Add to the bowl of mint, etc.
- Chop the Italian parsley. Add to the bowl of mint, etc.
- Chop the curly parsley. Add to the bowl of mint, etc.

- Add the pine nuts to the bowl of mint leaves, etc. Mix ingredients together. Set aside.
- In a separate bowl, put in the black pepper, sea salt, olive oil, lemon juice. Mix together.
- Pour the olive oil mixture over the cucumber mixture. Mix all ingredients together well.
- Serve immediately.

Snack Recipes

Avacado Mango Salsa

This recipe makes 2 servings and takes about 25 minutes of preparation.

What's in It

- Olive oil (3 tablespoons)
- Red onion (0.25 cup)
- Lime juice, fresh (2 tablespoons)
- Sea salt (1 teaspoon)
- Garlic, fresh (3 cloves)
- Cilantro, fresh (0.5 cup)
- Jalapeno pepper
- Tomatoes, medium (4 tomatoes)
- Avocado (1 avacado)
- Mango (1 mango)

How It's Made

- Chop the red onion. Put into a bowl.
- Mince the garlic. Put into the bowl with the red onion.
- Chop the cilantro. Put into the bowl with the red onion and garlic.
- De-seed and mince the jalapeno pepper. Put into the bowl with the onion, etc.
- Dice the tomatoes. Put into the bowl with the onion, etc.
- Peel, pit and dice the avocado. Put into the bowl with the onion, etc.
- Peel, de-seed and dice the mango. Put into the bowl with the onion, etc.
- Mix all ingredients together. Enjoy!

Traditional Hummus

This recipe makes 2–4 servings and takes about 10 minutes of preparation.

What's in It

- Sea salt (to taste)
- Cumin (1 teaspoon)
- Garlic (1 clove)
- Lemon juice (0.25 cup)
- Olive oil (1 tablespoon)
- Sesame seeds, raw (0.25 cup)
- Garbanzo beans (2 cans)

How It's Made

- Peel the garlic. Put into blender.
- Open cans of garbanzo beans.
- Reserve .25 cup of the liquid and pour it into the blender.
- Rinse the garbanzo beans and put the beans into the blender.
- Put all of the remaining ingredients into the blender. Blend.
- Add more water and/or olive oil slowly until you have reached the desired consistency.

Kale Chips

This recipe makes 1–2 servings and takes about 20 minutes of preparation.

What's in It

- Sea salt (0.25 teaspoon)
- Lemon juice (1 tablespoon)
- Grapeseed oil (2 tablespoons)
- Kale (1 bunch)

How It's Made

- Preheat oven to 350 degrees.
- Put the sea salt, lemon juice and grapeseed oil into a bowl. Mix together.
- Chop kale into 0.5-inch pieces. Add to the bowl.
- Massage the ingredients into the kale with your hands.
- Line a baking sheet using paper parchment.
- Turn out the ingredients onto the baking sheet.
- Bake for 12 minutes.

Just a Note About These Recipes

Intermittent fasting allows the body to heal itself and to get stronger, and it is important to make wise food choices for the hours that you do eat. These 20 recipes will help you create quality meals, salads, side dishes, and snack foods that provide the necessary daily nutrients and energy. Breakfast recipes were omitted since it will likely be breakfast that you will skip.

For the most part, these recipes omit refined sugar, hydrogenated oils, processed grains and other white food, pasteurized dairy, processed meat, conventional eggs, and artificial sweeteners.

That being the case, you are also eating what you need to eat if you rid your body of *candida overgrowth* or *parasite infestation*, which you read about in the chapter about hunger.

These particular recipes also help you to create dishes that allow the body to heal the digestive tract in persons who suffer from a condition that is commonly referred to as *leaky gut syndrome.*

The small intestines of a person with a leaky gut allow small particles of various things to get into the bloodstream, which causes various health problems over time. Some of the symptoms for leaky gut are the same for candida and for parasites.

The symptoms for leaky gut include the following:

- Food sensitivities
- Fatigue
- Anxiety and depression
- Constipation
- Hashimoto's Disease
- Obesity
- Lung tumors
- Skin problems
- Thyroid problems
- Colon problems
- Irritable bowel syndrome
- Crone's Disease
- Diarrhea
- Adrenal problems
- Kidney problems
- Frequent colds

If you have not heard of candida, parasites, or leaky gut, you are not alone. The medical establishment knows there is no money for them when patients are prescribed a few simple changes to their diets instead of a lifetime of pharmaceuticals.

Even if you just want to eat healthy food, these foods give you a natural diet, and everyone can benefit from eating foods that optimize metabolism, boost immune function, and lower inflammation.

Some of the recipes may be different than the recipe ingredients you are used to, but you will most likely be pleasantly surprised by how the food you create with them tastes and how they make you feel and look.

Conclusion

I hope this book was able to help you to learn about intermittent fasting and how you can lose weight by adopting it. My goal has always been to add value and improve your life.

Did you know that only 10% of the people who buy books get past the first chapter? If you made it this far, it shows you you're committed to making a change and pursuing your goals! I'm very proud of you.

If you enjoyed reading this book, or you learned a few things and find it helpful, then I'd like a favour from you: would you be kind enough to leave a review for this book on Amazon with a few kind words? I would be very grateful.

If you have any questions regarding Intermittent Fasting or Health and Fitness please send me a message at imdanieljonas@gmail.com. I'm here to help you!

Thank you and good luck!

Warmly,

Daniel Jonas